Ab Workouts
For Skinny Guys
Who Want To Build Some Muscle
and Turn Some Heads
Even If You've Never Been Able to Do That
With Other Workout Programs

Ab Exercises Series

Michael Weston

Edited by: Joyce Zborower

Ab Workouts for Skinny Guys Who Want to Build Some Muscle and Turn Some Heads Even If You've Never Been Able to do That With Other Workout Programs

Michael Weston

ISBN = 1497511542
ISBN-13 = 978-1497511545

Table of Contents

Ab Workouts
For Skinny Guys
Who Want To Build Some Muscle
and Turn Some Heads
Even If You've Never Been Able To Do That
With Other Workout Programs

Body Building Routines to Build Muscle Fast (But Safely!)

Anyone starting body building routines with the goal of building muscle mass naturally wants to get there fast. But one of the major reasons newbies tend to drop out right away is injury… from trying to build muscle mass too quickly. There is a way out of that dilemma.

First, be honest about where you're starting from and what you can achieve within the first three months. Some people hike, bike, or do other activities for fun that help keep their bodies in shape. They can start at a higher level than those who've been couch potatoes for years.

Second, rest assured that you can build muscle mass to your desired level within 6-12 months. Done correctly, you'll see initial results much sooner. But your goal is, or at least should be, a long-term commitment to a regular workout program and proper diet. Persistence – and the proper techniques – are the keys to success.

Tips to Safely Build Muscle Fast

Before we talk about those, here are some preliminary tips. Be sure you start with a weight that you can lift without excess exertion about 10-15 times. That helps avoid injury and gives you the feeling you can do what's needed. Use proper form, including breathing right. And, truly important: stay hydrated. Correct fluid levels are vital for muscle and overall health.

Here are **two body building routines** to get you started on that road to better health, and a more attractive you…

Squats

The squat will really help you build those large muscle groups fast. That gives you visible results in the shortest possible time because it works more muscle fibers and works them harder.

Prepare a barbell with the proper weight, as discussed above. Support the bar on the shoulder blades. Keep your elbows beneath the wrists. Stand about shoulder width with your feet placed in a natural position, pointed slightly outwards.

Now, squat — i.e. bend the knees, slowly, making sure to keep your balance. Beginners should always use a spotter for safety. Keep your spine slightly curved inward, not rounded outward (like a turtle). Move down like you were about to sit on a sofa, but don't overdo it. Don't extend the knees very much beyond the toes. Keep most of the weight back on the heels to really work those quadriceps.

Chin-Ups

The traditional chin-up requires no weights, so it's a great natural body building routine to help you build muscle mass fast and safely. You can use a bar in a door frame inside the house (just make sure it's screwed in securely enough to be able to hold your weight without pulling free), or the local playground (after hours, with permission), at the gym… anywhere.

They're really simple. Just grasp the bar above your head and pull your body up slowly (no jerking), then lower yourself slowly. For effective results you need to have the bar high enough so that your feet rise at least six inches off the ground. At least twelve inches is preferable. For a variation, you can purchase sand-filled ankle or waist straps to add extra difficulty, but work up to this.

Perform your bodybuilding routines regularly. Mon-Tue, rest on Wed, Thu-Fri, rest on the weekend is one good way to go. Rest allows the body to recuperate and gives it time to rebuild those stressed muscle fibers, which makes them bigger and stronger. That's how you build muscle fast, and safely.

Build Muscle Fast

It's About The Right Foods And Proper Exercises

If your dream is to build up your muscles, then you may be interested in finding out how to build muscle fast. Being knowledgeable about what it takes to build muscle fast can be very helpful when deciding which exercises to include in your workouts. Are you wanting to do sports? … Are you hoping to look great at the beach? … Well, whatever your reason, there is a right way and a wrong way to do it.

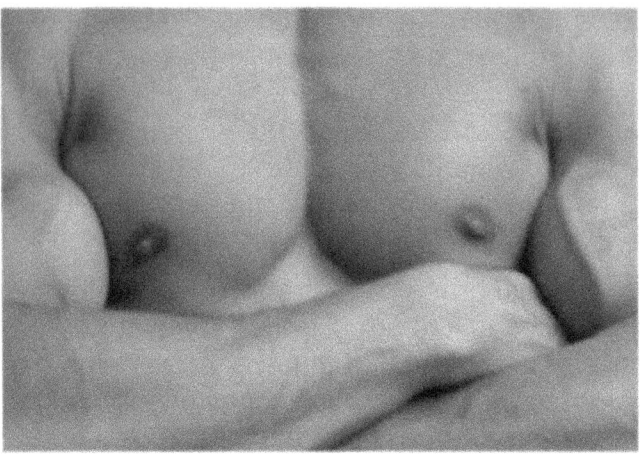

What NOT To Do

One common mistake that many people who are new to trying to get fit is to emulate the steps that professional bodybuilders perform in order to build up their muscles. They generally end up feeling overwhelmed and frustrated and inadequate.

Another mistake is to try to build muscle fast by going out and buying a lot of expensive workout equipment. It takes up a lot of space in their home and – usually – just ends up collecting dust.

To Build Muscle Fast, Start Slow

There is no magic bullet. The real solution to building muscle fast consists of two fundamental steps: (1) eat the correct foods, and (2) work out regularly using the correct exercises that specifically target your particular problem areas.

These two steps will ensure that you can build your muscle safely and naturally. To build muscle fast successfully, often you need do nothing more than eat well, exercise properly … and maybe also do some weight training.

If you elect to do the weight training, it's preferable that you choose to use free weights as opposed to depending on machines because using free weights allows your body to perform natural lifting movements. The use of machines, however, causes you to make unnatural motions that can lead to unnecessary injuries.

Also, a barbell or two can prove to be far more effective in helping you build muscle fast than all that expensive equipment. There are also many different natural exercise options available that spending extra money on a lot of equipment just isn't necessary.

Concentrate On Large Muscle Groups

When trying to build your muscles and get fit, start by concentrating your efforts on the large muscle groups rather than the smaller specific areas. Isolation exercises are great, but working on the large muscle groups will have a more noticeable effect on your whole body.

Eat A Healthy Diet

The role played by a healthy and proper diet in your muscle building plan cannot be overemphasized. Eating the right foods (your fuel) will facilitate better weight training and simplify the whole process of losing body fat, gaining muscle, getting fit, and looking better.

Supplements can play a role in a healthy diet. Many people consume supplements to help create better and bigger biceps. One that's recommended for this is L-glutamine.

Bottom Line

The bottom line with regard to learning how to build muscle fast is: In case the results you're looking for don't show up immediately, don't panic and don't give up!
As long as you

(1) eat the right foods
(2) continue to do your workouts regularly, and
(3) keep a record of your activities and progress
you will begin to see results – and probably sooner rather than later.

Build Muscle Fast and Burn Fat... The Wrong Way

For an area where science — or at least common sense — should be king, there is a lot of voodoo published about bodybuilding, nutrition, and related subjects. If you want to build muscle fast and burn fat while building it, a little knowledge — and forgetting the hype — goes a long way.

Forget fad diets, complicated nutrition timing, and much of the rest of modern muscle building and fat burning advice (which will be changed three months after you read it). The long and short of it — and nutrition science has known this for decades — is that if you burn more calories than you consume you will lose weight. Keep losing, and you will burn fat.

The body stores fat in the first place because we've evolved to not expect a meal every few hours. Once the available sugars are used up the body will release stored fat and burn it for energy. There are some ways to be more efficient about that, for sure, but that's the basic idea.

So, here's the right way to build muscle fast.

So, what kinds of body building routines will help you build muscle fast and burn fat — in order to lose weight, look great, and be healthy? Their number and variety are legion. But for truly fast fat burning and muscle building, working large muscle groups really helps. It stands to reason that the more muscle fibers involved, the more energy is required to work them.

Fortunately, that gives you an incredibly long and varied list from which to choose. You can focus on your quadriceps and hamstrings one day — both large muscles that take a lot of the body's energy quota to keep them moving during a hard workout. Then, you can let them rest, and work on another group another day, say, the lats (the back muscles along the sides of your body that make people 'triangular').

Certainly, most body building routines will work a wide range of muscles/muscle groups, even when they're not the focus. Your abs may be the focus when you do sit-ups, but you can't help working the calves, or even your sterno(s) (the neck muscles in front) at the same time. Chin-ups will work the lats, pecs, and deltoids hardest, but you can't avoid doing good for your biceps and triceps during the exercise.

The reason, once again though, to focus on those larger muscles is to really build muscle fast, in order to see results soonest. Most novices get discouraged when they don't see weight loss, toning, more bulk, and the other benefits right away.

At the same time, with a good diet that includes the right balance of protein, carbs, and healthy fats, you can burn unwanted fat. Nutritional balance that contains all the essential compounds — and that avoids an excess of those things we all love so much — is key.

It's important not to expect too much, too soon from your muscle building/fat burning routines and diet. But you can achieve visible results within a few months, if you stick with it.

Building Muscle without Weights

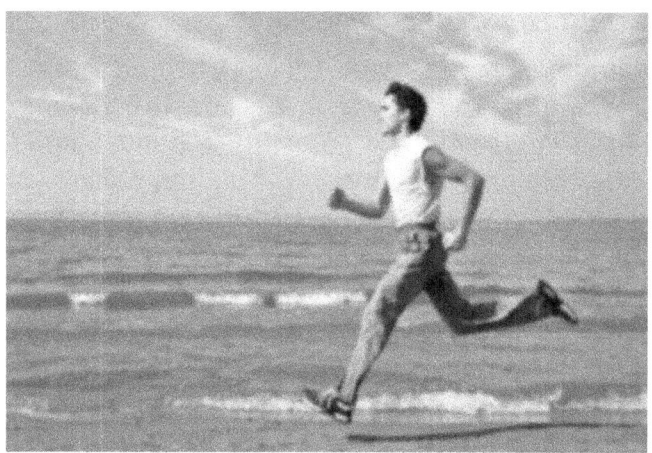

There are dozens of effective ways to build muscle mass
without weights. Sometimes it's even more efficient. It's
certainly more convenient — no trips to the gym — and can be
safer, too. It's not an either/or proposition, either. You can do
both and get the unique benefits of each body building
approach.

Consider the simple, traditional push-up. Do them the
traditional way and you'll get some cardio benefit and help
build your biceps, triceps, and back muscles (lats) to a certain
degree. But to really increase their size and clearly define
them you need weights, right?

Not necessarily. Anything that makes the muscles involved in
push-ups work harder will necessarily stimulate blood flow and
the growth of muscle proteins in the body. Here are just a few
ways to do that.

Change the angle of your body. Instead of lying with your feet on the floor, put them on a chair, a footstool, the couch, the steps of your deck… anywhere safe and stable. Gravity then requires you to exert extra force to raise your torso by the same amount you would normally. Simple, no?

The results will speak for themselves. You'll get well-defined biceps and bigger pecs if you stick to a regular routine. You can work your way up, and make it even tougher, by gradually increasing that angle. Then, for a variation, try those same push-ups with only one arm at a time.

The same technique can be used to enhance the effectiveness of sit-ups. Ordinary sit-ups help burn calories, as well as define and strengthen your abdominals, glutes, and lats. Working those large muscles (not the only ones that get a workout, of course) helps you achieve that great look you want to impress the ladies and feel good. Work them harder and get more of those muscle-mass building and weight loss benefits. Here's how…

Instead of doing the classic "lie flat on your back on a level surface with your toes under the couch, put your hands behind your head…," vary the method.

One helpful variation is simply, again, to change the angle. Select a comfortable, smooth surface that's at an angle. That could be an incline board. Or, you could seek out a slanted sidewalk and use a mat. Find a smooth stretch of grass on a hill. Then do your normal number of reps and sets.

Another variation involves giving your abs less help in moving your head to your knees. Simply keep your hands at your sides, with palms facing down on the ground. Or, straighten out your legs. Simple, classic, effective. And no weights required.

Want to get a great cardio workout, one that also builds muscle in your quadriceps, without using weights? Equally easy. Here again, the idea is to make it harder to perform the exercise. Instead of cushy grass, pick a more resistant surface.

Beach sand works great for this. It makes it harder to run, but still provides all the cushion you need to keep your muscles, joints, and connective tissue from getting overstressed. Running along the beach, especially near the water line, is great for this. Then work up to dry sand, which is even tougher. Try it in a foot of water beyond the shoreline and you'll see how tough working in wet can really be, though.

Don't have a beach nearby? Visit your local volleyball court. Go to a kids playground (when the kids aren't around) and run in circles. Seek out the local golf course, off hours or on days the golfers aren't around, and alternate running over grass with running over the sand pits.

Building muscle to peak performance and peak form without weights is simple. Just increase the force required (which is what the weights do, after all) more than the standard method. Change the angle, change the surface, change your technique. Get the results: a great looking you.

Great Muscle Diet Guidelines — for everyone

You're sticking to a regular workout to build muscle mass fast and burn fat. Great. Exercise is essential, but good nutrition is vital for overall health, as well as looking and feeling good.

Now is the right time to fold in that second all-important aspect: the right muscle diet.

You know you're supposed to be eating low-fat protein, so you've made skinless chicken a regular part of your diet. Excellent. But did you know that getting too little fat can also be a problem?

Fats are essential for a wide range of natural body processes, including good nerve development and helping the body create certain essential compounds. Lean beef — far from being the evil food it was once depicted — is a great source of muscle building protein with a good balance of fat.

Red meat not only has the protein you need to build muscle (muscles themselves are protein, after all). It also contains creatine, vitamins, and vital minerals. Protein you consume is broken down by the body into amino acids, which are then re-combined into human proteins – including the type that compose muscle fibers.

White meat is also good, though, and none better than fish. Tuna is a good source of protein and omega-3 fatty acids, but with lower levels than salmon. Try both for variety.

Omega-3 fatty acids are essential but the body doesn't produce them internally. All it needs must come from outside. They help with brain health and keeping the immune system in good working order. Make them a regular part of your muscle building diet.

Other muscle building foods include various kinds of carbs. Carbohydrates often get a bad rep because people associate them with sugars (which they essentially resemble). But remember that sugar or carbs are the body's basic energy battery. Without them, all cellular processes would come to a halt quickly.

Still, there are carbs and there are carbs. Ease off on the pasta (good in moderation and a great source of fiber) and try some spaghetti squash instead. Veggies are good, as everyone knows. This helps you turn consuming a needed aspect of nutrition from a chore to a delight.

You've read that yogurt is good for you, and you read right. The lactobacillus acidophilus and natural additives in modern yogurts are a good way to boost your digestive system health. Among other things it helps create Vitamin K. That is an important aid to your muscle building diet.

Well, do yourself a favor and try some fat-free Greek yogurt. Greek yogurt has none of the added sugar that some commercial brands add to make up for the blandness that can accompany non-fat foods. This style is creamier and tangier, so no sugar needed. It also has twice the protein and half the carbs of 'normal' yogurt. Add colored fruit, such as raspberries or blueberries, for flavor and to get those really helpful phytonutrients.

A muscle diet contains muscle building foods with muscle building protein. Lucky for you, those also happen to be foods that form a great part of a highly nutritious and tasty diet for general health. Win-win, as they say.

How to Burn Fat Fast

If you want to learn how to burn fat fast, you need to speed up your metabolism. And to speed up your metabolism, you have to:
(1) eat the right kinds and amounts of food at the proper time of day
(2) work out regularly using appropriate exercises

So let's talk about each of these areas and find out exactly what's involved.

Eating Right

The first thing to know about eating right is that starving yourself is just as harmful to your body as stuffing yourself is. In other words, you have to eat to live but you don't have to live to eat! …i.e., don't eat so much that you become uncomfortable – like after a Thanksgiving dinner.

You should always time your meals so that you eat before you begin craving food. If you follow this simple convention, your metabolism will help you. This is how to burn fat fast and you'll also be eating less because you'll feel full faster. There really is no need to finish everything on your plate just because it's on your plate. Stop eating when you're full.

Eat your largest meal in the morning as this provides fuel for doing your day's tasks.

Don't eat right before going to bed because your metabolism slows down when you go to bed and your food won't get digested very well.

Eliminate refined white sugar, refined white flour, and added salt from your diet. Instead, eat plenty of fresh fruits, vegetables, whole grains and proteins. There are also healthy fats and not so healthy fats. Eat the healthy ones like olive oil, avocados, etc.

Speaking of fats, many professionals recommend eating low-fat-this or low-fat-that. Personally, I don't think that's a good idea because when the food manufacturer takes out something, it usually alters the taste of the food so, to compensate, they usually add sugar. If you've learned how to burn fat fast, you now know that added sugar is not something you need in your diet.

Work Out Regularly

Another facet of learning how to burn fat fast is doing cardio exercises regularly. The smart way to do cardio is 30 minutes in the morning and 30 minutes in the evening. Research has shown that breaking up your sessions like this will help you lose more fat more quickly than if you were to regularly do a 60 minute cardio workout.

Replacing body fat with muscle mass will also help you burn fat fast. Do exercises that stimulate muscle growth. Adding more muscle will help speed up your metabolism and help burn fat because your body will naturally burn more calories – even when you're resting.

Is a Burning Fat Diet Right for You?

Dedication!

An ominous word, isn't it? But that's what you'll need if you want to stay on a burning fat diet. It's not easy to say "NO" to all the yummy things you've been used to putting in your mouth. 'Getting on' a burning fat diet is one thing; 'STAYING ON' is something else.

Or, even if you believe you already do say no to a lot of stuff and think your diet is pretty healthy right now, you have to realize that when you make a conscious, concerted effort to make your diet very strict and are very cautious about what you swallow — this is when you finally realize just how hard it is.

Whether we believe it or not, most of us are already addicted to sugar by the time we're two or three years old. This is because baby food manufacturers add sugar to their products to make them taste better to the mothers who sample the food before they feed it to their babies.

Breaking a sugar addiction is tough. Doable, but tough. But it's one of the most important things you can do for yourself if you're really serious about being on a burning fat diet. Sugary foods can add to your body fat. (If you want a reference to some material that will help you break a sugar addiction, use the 'Contact Me' form with the subject line "Break sugar addiction reference", and I'll send it right out to you.

Salt is the other major bug-a-boo.

If you decide that a burning fat diet is right or you, then you'll need to seriously control those salty foods as well that give you that uncomfortable bloated feeling by making your body retain fluids.

This is especially important during the summertime because summer is a great time for snacking on pretzels and soda and/or beer at those backyard cookouts.

Now, if you want to go on a burning fat diet, in addition to cutting out salt and refined sugar, there are a few other things that you'll want to keep in mind as well.

Fruits and Vegetables

You may not be aware of just how major a role fruits and vegetables play in the human diet. Few people are.

But if you want to be successful with your burning fat diet, then you'll want to find the best burning fat diet available out there — one that's going to have you eating more fruits and vegetables. Especially the dark green leafy vegetables that are so important for increasing your fiber.

If possible, eat your fruits in the morning. Fruits have some natural sugars in them (which are not nearly as harmful as refined sugars) so if you eat them in the morning your body has time to turn those sugars into energy instead of body fat.

Fresh, clean water is extremely important. No matter what kind of diet you decide to follow — a burning fat diet or something else — make sure your water is as free of harmful chemicals (chlorine, fluoride, etc.) and other contaminants as possible.

Few people are drinking as much water as their body actually needs. The recommended amount is six to eight (6 – 8) glasses per day. Drinking 6 – 8 glasses of water per day will also help you burn fat because thirst sometimes disguises itself as hunger. If you think you're hungry — but instead of eating food, drink water — you might just find you're feeling full again.

These are all great tips that will help you burn fat, get in the best shape of your life, and stay that way for the rest of your life.

The 6 Pack Abs Diet Plan: What You Need to Know

It's understandable why we all want to have 6 pack abs, but they don't just happen by wishing and expecting your body will change all by itself.

If you want to get a really great looking washboard stomach, then you're going to have to come up with a great 6 pack abs diet plan along with the proper exercise program that will get you where you want to go.

Of course the actual exercising that you do will be the most important determining factor in whether or not you'll get the body you want because without the proper exercises on the specific target areas that need changing and strengthening, you'll never be able to see those 6 pack abs. But the 6 pack diet plan is also vital to your success.

People don't generally realize just how important a role their diet plays on the way they feel and look. A steady diet of fast food and diet drinks can undermine just about any good exercise program.

Only by following a proper 6 pack abs diet plan will you be able to get in shape, target those abdominal muscles with the proper exercises and finally see the difference this will make in the way you feel and look.

Creating Your Diet Plan

A one-size-fits-all diet plan that stops there won't work. Customization. That's the key to a really effective 6 pack abs diet plan that will work. Your plan has to be specific for your individual nutritional needs.

Eating healthy is not an option: it's a requirement. But the very first thing you need to do is make a list of
– (1) any foods you are allergic to
– (2) foods you don't like the taste of and just can't stand to eat
– (3) and so on.

Now that you have your list of basic foods that you don't want to eat or can't have included in you 6 pack abs diet plan, it's time to start customizing your diet. This starting point is figuring out all the different types of foods that you can and should be eating.

So for your 6 pack abs diet plan, your main focus should be on including different kinds of fruits and vegetables. These are natural foods that contain a lot of fiber (which is good for your bowels) and don't contain high fats or sugars (which is good for your body because they don't contribute to body fat).

Just make sure that you try to eat the fruit in the earlier part of the day — breakfast and morning snack, in a smoothie for inst

ance — so that your body has a chance to use the natural sugars in the fruit for energy for the better part of the day.

Your 6 Pack Abs Workout: what you need to know

To get the most benefit from your 6 pack abs workout, you need to pay attention to three different but related areas if you want your body to show maximum response to the actual exercises. These areas are:

... (1) diet

... (2) cardio

... (3) building muscle with specific exercises

So, let's briefly cover each of these areas.

The Right Diet for Your 6 Pack Abs Workout

The old adage "You can't out-train a bad diet," is absolutely true. Regularly eating a junk-food/fast-food diet will undo all your efforts in the gym. Also, when you eat your largest meal of the day is also important. Most of us eat our largest meal at night – when we're least active.

Your biggest meal should be eaten in the morning. Food is your body's fuel just like gas is fuel for your car. Give your body the fuel it needs early in the day so that you have the extra energy you need for your cardio and 6 pack abs workout. This also gives your body the opportunity to to burn off the calories instead of storing them as fat while you sleep.

The best 6 pack abs workout diet contains a lot of natural foods like fresh fruits, vegetables and whole grains. It should also be a customized meal plan for your particular needs and tastes. Natural foods have more of the nutrients that your body requires to burn fat and build muscle. Muscle building also depends on an adequate intake of protein which includes red meat, fish and beans.

Cardio – to lose that Belly Fat

Cardio 6 pack abs workout exercises exercise your heart muscle and increase your heart rate. You should plan on doing cardio exercises at least 20 minutes per day, 5 days per week. Jogging, swimming, and cycling are all popular ways of having fun while giving your heart the exercise it needs. As your body becomes comfortable with this program, increase the time allotted to it.

Your 6 Pack Abs Workout Muscle Building Technique

Here I will share two introductory workouts you can use to begin to develop that washboard stomach that everybody wants. Start with 2 sets of 20 reps (for both exercises), 5 days per week. Each week, add one more set.

1. CRUNCHES – lie flat on your back with your knees bent and your hands behind your head. Use your abdominal muscles to pull your upper body off the floor. Hold this position while you slowly count to 5, keep your abs tight, slowly lower your body, repeat.

2. BICYCLE CRUNCHES – Lie flat on your back with your legs set apart at a 45° angle and your hands behind your head. Slowly bring one knee toward your chest while at the same time bringing your elbow on your other side towards your knee. Reverse. You should feel somewhat like you're peddling a bicycle.

The Best Way to Lose Belly Fat Naturally: A Few Tips

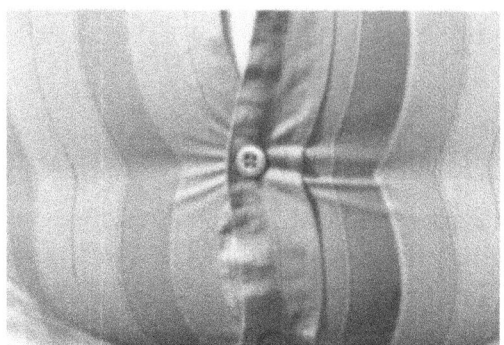

Excess belly fat makes your life difficult in many ways:
– it's hard to reach you feet to tie your shoes
– sometimes you can't even see your feet
– it's difficult to find clothes that fit and look good
– excess belly fat increases your chances for a heart attack
– it could even be a factor in your lack of a romantic relationship

And despite your best efforts, it is very difficult to make unattractive, stubborn, excess belly fat go away.

So if you're interested in knowing the best way to lose belly fat naturally so you can look and feel better, there are two things you need to do:

#1 – Change Your Eating Habits!

Easier said than done. But the very best way to lose belly fat naturally is to start by changing your eating habits to include healthier natural foods, exclude fast-food junk foods, and at the same time.....

#2 – Engage in some form of regular exercise.

We'll talk about #1 here.

There are certain diet plans that have proven to be effective in helping people lose that unwanted belly fat. If you're really serious, you might want to take a look at the one I'm recommending:

Another diet tip for the best way to lose belly fat naturally is to make sure you're eating sufficient protein every day. Protein provides a number of benefits for someone who's trying to lose belly fat naturally. It helps to keep your blood glucose levels normal which helps to control your insulin levels — good for controling or preventing diabetes. It increases your rate of metabolism and helps to burn fat. Also, by eating sufficient protein, you're giving your body what it needs in order to build muscle tissue.

Whole grains in your diet are a whole lot better for you than refined grains. Whole grains help increase muscle tone.

Some people will tell you to stop eating grains altogether because they are primarily carbohydrate and carbohydrate is a kind of sugar which your body can use to turn into fat. Bad idea! Carbohydrate is brain food. Without sufficient carbohydrate in your diet, your brain doesn't work very well.

The types of carbohydrate that should be eliminated from your diet are the REFINED carbohydrates. An easy way to remember what not to eat is: If it's white, dont eat it. …white flour …white sugar …white salt. … and that includes those foods that include this 'white stuff' as ingredients.

Eating fresh fruit and vegetables is also considered another best wat to lose belly fat naturally, as is including lean meats in your meal plans.

If possible however, avoid processed foods. This includes foods that are sold as "diet foods" and "low fat foods". They are all adulterated and not good for you because when manufacturers take out something, they generally put in extra sugar. You don't need to be eating extra sugar.

Natural Bodybuilding Workout Routines For A Great Look

Maybe you're what's called a hardgainer. You've tried and tried to gain muscle mass — working out daily, following expert advice, and taking tons of supplements. Yet, you're still underweight, maybe even scrawny, and with poor definition. What to do?

You could go overboard and start working out like the pros. You might even be tempted to start taking anabolic steroids to pump up. But you're concerned about side effects and have been reading about an alternative, one called natural bodybuilding. Again, what to do?

First, do yourself a favor. Get good and scared by reading up on all the dangers of long-term steroid use. Then, get disappointed when you consider who writes all the expert advice you've read in fitness magazines. It comes from writers hired by the companies that own supplement makers... who also own the magazines.

Ready to start fresh in your approach now? Thought so.

Fortunately, you can build muscle mass with natural bodybuilding routines, and often quicker than you might think. You can look great with your shirt off, and attract all the women you could ever want. Or, at least all the ones you could make time for. No drugs. No monthly supplement budget that could pay for trips to Cabo. Just safe, natural workout routines that get you ripped and looking good.

Here are just two examples to get you started on that body you've always wanted, but never quite could achieve. As you read them, keep in mind that one key is to work those large muscle groups, such as those of the back, pecs, and so forth. That's where you get the most gain for your efforts.

Bench Press

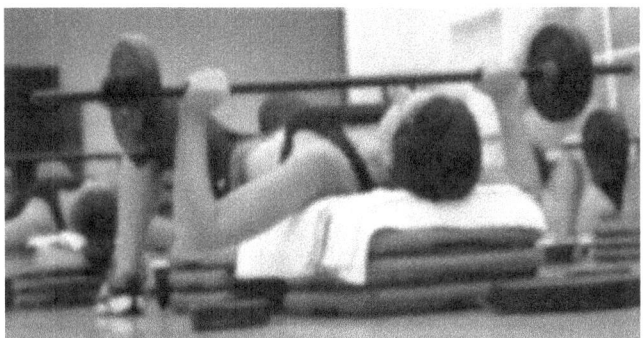

The classic bench press helps work more muscle fibers because it engages your pecs, triceps, deltoids, and biceps all at once. It's simple. Lie on a flat bench and plant your feet flat on the floor about shoulder width.

Now, with your hands placed about shoulder width apart, hold the barbell above your body and lower it slowly to the middle of your chest. Be sure not to bounce the weight off your chest. Do 10 reps, rest and repeat 3 times.

Standing Military Press

Here's another traditional exercise that remains one of the best for building those large muscle groups that help you bulk up without becoming bulky. Stand with your feet about shoulder width apart and lock your legs. Let the barbell rest comfortably in your hands at chest height. Keep your elbows under the bar and slanted slightly inward.

Now, press the bar overhead by extending your arms all the way. No need to jerk; in fact, you should avoid it. You want to do this smoothly at moderate speed. Now lower to chin height, or even a little lower, down to your chest. Do whatever feels comfortable. Do 10 reps, rest and repeat 3 times.

No one can give a universal recommendation for what weight to start with for these bodybuilding workout routines. It depends on where you're starting from. For some real newbies trying to build muscle mass for the first time, 30 lbs might be as much as can be safely handled. For others, 50 lbs or even 100 lbs is the right place to start. Start low and build up as you gain confidence.

Natural bodybuilding lets you gain muscle mass fast, yet safely, without the use of harmful steroids or useless supplements.

"Finally Get Those 6 Pack Abs You've Been Dreaming About and Turn Some Heads!"

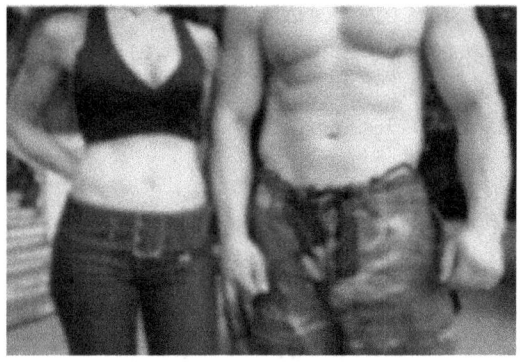

6 Pack Abs for Guys & Gals

So you've decided to go after hot muscles fast, i.e. 6 pack abs.

You've chosen a difficult goal. However, getting 6 pack abs is not an impossible goal, but you'll have to have a certain amount of drive and determination — and it probably won't seem that fast.

Working out to tone up any part of your body is never easy. The only way to get those hot muscles fast is to put in the time and effort and stick with it until you reach your goal.

Going after 6 pack abs is painful. The exercises make your muscles burn and sting. Those are the times you'll need to push through and just keep going because that's when you will be getting the best results.

Now if you really want those hot muscles fast, you'll have to pay attention to a few more things besides just determination and motivation.

Here's How You Do It

First, to get 6 pack abs you need to change your diet.

You have to start saying "NO" to fast food, sodas, salty foods, and snacky stuff that has no nutritional value. These are the foods that contain the highest amounts of refined white flour, refined white sugar, and white salt. A good rule of thumb is: If it's white, don't eat it. This will probably be the hardest thing you've ever done so far in you life.

And you'll have to start saying "YES" to healthier choices such as fresh fruits and vegetables, whole grains, and clear clean fresh water as your beverage of choice.

Go through your cupboards and get rid of everything you shouldn't put in your mouth. …unless of course you're living with other people. Then you'll have to take their needs into consideration and just be more vigilant with your own food choices.

Now, if you truly want to get 6 pack abs and develop hot muscles fast, another thing you'll have to do is get more active. Eating the right kinds of foods will help, and that's great and will help in the weight-loss department, but if you're not exercising properly and specifically working on your most serious problem areas, you won't be able to get those beautiful 6 pack abs.

Though your workouts need to exercise and tone your whole body, your main focus should be on tightening, toning and strengthening your abdominal muscles.

There are many different kinds of exercises that work well for this. The best idea, however, is for you to create your own workout plan with exercises tailored to your particular problem areas that you're comfortable sticking with and doing over and over and over.

That's how you'll make your quickest and best progress in developing your 6 pack abs and hot muscles fast.

"What's The Best Abdominal Routine?"

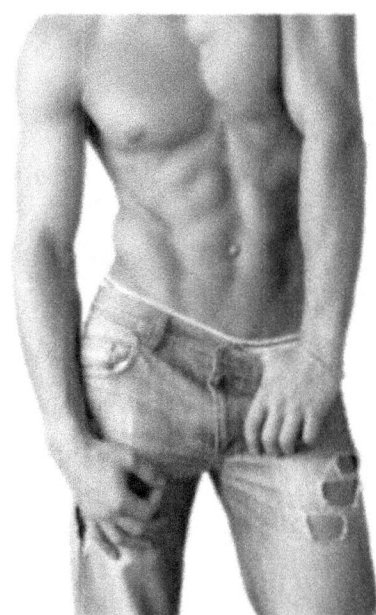

There is no single best abdominal routine.

There are, however, a number of exercises that specifically target the abdominal muscles and that are geared towards helping you get those 6 pack abs that everybody wants. Ideally, your personal trainer will choose the best abdominal routine for you that will target your specific problem areas. S/he will also be able to expertly direct you and teach the significance of preciseness of execution once you become familiar with the basic movements.

The best abdominal routine design will also include a customized meal-plan/dietary-recommendations-plan that stresses high quality proteins, composite carbohydrates, and healthy fats that will greatly assist you in maintaining your intense training program.

Simple Abdominal Exercises

Your best abdominal routine will consist
of exercises recommended by strength and fitness professionals because their experience with numerous people over many years has shown them what works and what doesn't.

So according to the professionals, the best abdominal routine starts with (1) Swiss Ball Ab Crunches followed by (2) Inverse Crunches and then ending with (3) Ab Crunches. These are to be done in 3 sets of 12 – 15 reps. Crunches help tone your muscles – but someone who's overweight has to lose the weight before they can see their muscles. This is the challenge of sticking with a fat-loss diet.

Even if you're not planning to go after 6 pack abs, strengthening your abdominal muscles is still important because strong abs reduce the risk of lower back injuries, help decrease low back pain if your back is already injured, and help to tone your whole torso.

From a trainer's point of view, the most efficient and best abdominal routine consists of: (1) ab crunches that bend the upper abdominal muscles and serve as the base for the whole workout, (2) inverse crunches that tone the lower abs, and

(3) side folds that work on exercising the sidelong oblique muscles. Also, the American Council on Exercise declared Bicycle Crunches to be among the best abdominal exercises because it uses every muscle in the abs to develop a well-built torso.

Exercising, eating well, and developing 6 pack abs is no mean deed. Uncovering those 6 pack abs needs constant checking of what, how much, and when one eats. Discipline and patience are definitely necessary.

However, it must be repeated that even the best abdominal routine may not make the splashboard abs you're hoping to see if you have a slow metabolism. But there are ways to quicken your metabolism such as (1) healthy snacking between meals, (2) eating low glycemic index carbohydrates, (3) aerobic or cardio exercises, (4) drinking adequate water to stay perked up, (5) lifting weights, and (6) checking your food consumption.

If you're able to strengthen your abdominal muscles, reduce your belly fat, and use a proven program that's already proven its effectiveness with others, your chances of developing those 6 pack abs is greatly increased.

What's the Best Ab Workout? Three Good Options

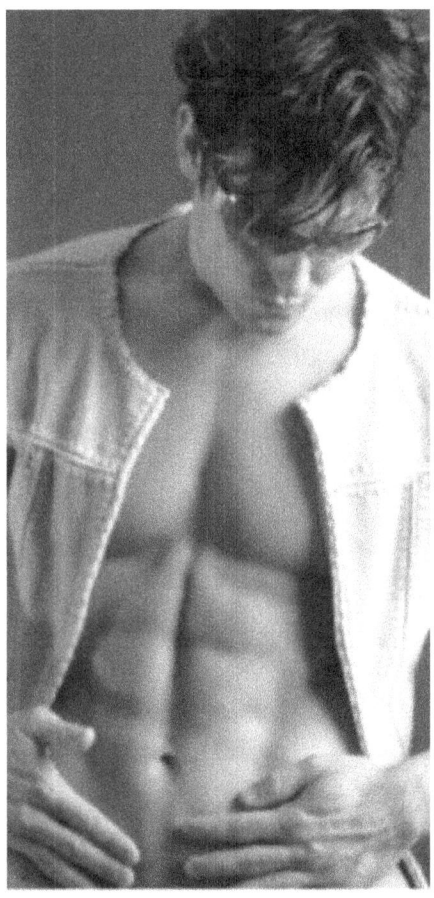

6 Pack Abs

Opinions may differ on just which is the best ab workout plan from the many available because there are so many to choose from. However, each one will do something different for you. So when choosing an ab workout plan it's important to know what benefit you're looking for and whether that plan is designed to provide that specific benefit.

For example, nobody wants a big belly. Not only is a big belly unattractive, a big belly is associated with heart problems.

And while everybody wants an improved, slim and strong abdomen, most workout plans are "one-size-fit-all". You need to discover the most effective **ab** workouts available — ones that provide the SPECIFIC benefits you're looking for that you'll actually be able to do.

For anyone interested, the key to finding the best ab workout (the one that's best FOR YOU) is to learn about the various routines and then choose one that suits your own specific abilities, needs and capabilities.

Whichever routine you choose, the best ab workout is the one that you'll stick with that will make your abdominal (stomach) muscles stiffer and stronger.

Crunches

Some would say that crunches are the best ab workout routine around, and why not? The only equipment you need is a mat to lay on.

To do crunches, start by learning to press your feet strongly to the floor. Then raise your knees and, with both hands placed behind your head, lift up your head without pulling at your neck in the process.

At the same time you're lifting your head, tighten your stomach muscles. (This is why this exercise is called 'cru8nches'!) Now maintain this position for a few short seconds — count to 5 — before releasing and returning to your original position.

A few repetitions (generally around 10 to start with) will get your body accustomed to one of the best ab workout options out there. As long as you can perform a consistent number of reps on a regular basis you will start to see results within just a few sessions.

Knee Ups

Another option for choosing the best ab workout is doing knee ups. These require sitting on a bench with both of your hands grasping each side of the bench. Then you need to extend your legs out in front of you — not touching the floor. Once fully extended, simply pull your knees back slowly toward your chest.

This movement will ensure proper contraction of your stomach muscles. By first maintaining this position for a few seconds and then releasing and repeating the same movements over again, you should be able, in a short amount of time, to develop the kind of attractive and strong abs that every male desires.

About 25 reps are all it takes, in sets of 3. For those who are new to this phrase, it means: Do the above 3 times. Rest for a few seconds. Then do it 3 more time. Rest. …etc. for 25 repetition.

Twists

Believe it or not, simple body twists aren't only considered effective, they're used so often by trainers they're considered one of the best ab workouts right along with the other two already mentioned. Body twists are probably a lot easier than the other two also.

To do simple body twists, stand up straight with your feet set slightly apart and your arms held in the air straight out from your shoulders at you sides.

Now, simply move your body slowly and deliberately from a facing-front position, twisting at your waist, toward your right until your arms are pointing directly in front and behind you. Hold this position while you slowly count to 5.

Slowly turn to a face-forward position (your original position) and the twist to your left until your arms are pointing directly in front of and behind you. Again, hold this position while you slowly count to 5 and then slowly move back to the face-forward position. That's all there is to it!

Doing a certain amount of reps on a regular basis of any one or a combination of these 3 options can improve your abs greatly and give you the attractive body that you're looking for. By trying them all, you'll find which option(s) work best you you.

So experiment and have fun!

"What's the Best Way to Lose Weight and Get In Shape?"

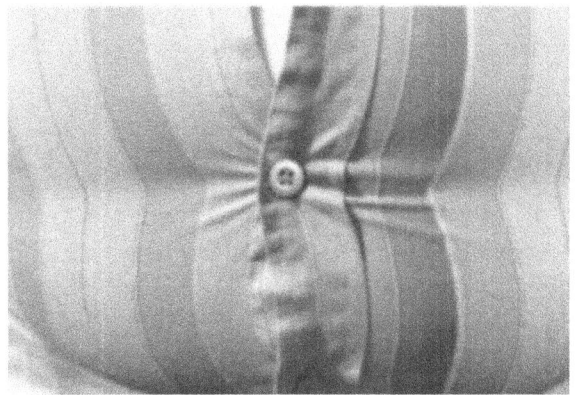

So, you want to know the best way to lose weight and get in shape. Losing weight means losing body fat. Getting in shape means replacing that body fat with lean muscle and exercising that muscle to make it more responsive, i.e. creating body tone.

The very best way to lose weight and get in shape requires a combination of the right diet while simultaneously doing the right exercises. Dieting alone won't get you the results you want; exercising alone won't do it, either. You need both –

together – at the same time. And you should also get yourself some help because will power alone won't do it, either.

Step 1: Get Help

You may never have cared about losing weight and getting in shape before. If this is the case, it's likely you don't have a clue how to begin. So start by getting yourself some help.

If you want to find out the best way to lose weight and get in shape, find somebody who's already done it – then find out what they did – then do it!

Step 2: Change Your Diet

A fast food/junk food diet will undo whatever benefits you get from your workouts. There's a saying, "You can't out-train a bad diet." It's true. So if you're really serious about finding and using the best way to lose weight and get in shape, ditch the junk and start eating natural foods like fresh fruits and vegetables and other foods that have a lot of good healthy nutrients.

To lose weight and get in shape, you need to be aware of the importance of what you're putting in your mouth. What you're eating will have a significant effect on your weight as well as the way you're feeling in general, so make sure you're eating healthy.

Step 3: Exercise

The third part of this puzzle has to do with replacing your body fat with muscle and then toning that muscle. Make sure you're working out on a regular basis doing exercises that are specifically targeting your most troublesome problem areas.

If you're not exercising, then you won't be able to get in shape. Dieting alone won't do it. It's just that simple – and that complicated.

How to Get 6 Pack Abs at 40

Who doesn't want to know how to get 6 pack abs at 40? Almost nobody, I would imagine.

So if you're one of the many who are interested in finding out about how you can get and keep 6 pack abs at 40, listen up because there are a few steps to this process and it's not easy.

Getting 6 pack abs at any age is never easy, but getting 6 pack abs at 40 or above is a special challenge. And if you also want that washboard stomach, you're going to have more trouble than you've ever imagined.

So if you're really serious about getting your body back in shape and really serious about having those 6 pack abs at 40, you will definitely want to keep reading and make sure you pay close attention to the rest of the information here.

Dedication and Motivation

The absolute keys to getting and keeping 6 pack abs at 40 or above are dedication and motivation.
– How badly do you want it?
– Why do you want it?
– What do you think your life will be like once you have it?
These are the questions you need to answer for yourself.
And those are the answers that will keep you going back to the gym — or not.

And once you've achieved your goal of 6 pack abs at 40, you'll need to maintain the dedication and motivation to stay in shape and stay healthy for the rest of your life.

Getting in Shape

Step 1: Clean Out Your Kitchen Cupboards!

What a silly first step for getting in shape. Right? Well, not really. Whether you've decided to go for the 6 pack abs or work on some of your body's other problem areas, the very first thing you need to do is throw out all the junk food in your cupboards! …before it ends up in your belly.

Of course, if you have other people also living in your house — like a spouse or kids — throwing out all the junk food may not be an option. Although you want them to eat healthy as well, arbitrarily making that kind of a decision for someone else is bound to cause trouble. So if you can't throw out the junk food physically, you can be extra careful about not putting it in your mouth.

Concentrate on eating the healthy foods like fruits and vegetables and whole grains in the forms of whole grain breads and cereals.

Step 2: Take the Time to Customize a Workout Plan for Yourself.

Whether you've decided to go after the 6 pack abs at 40 or work on other problem areas, you'll need to begin a regular exercise program to get back in shape.

When customizing your workout plan, you'll want to focus on your abdominal muscles. There are a lot of great exercises you can do that target your abs and reduce belly fat.

You'll want to put your main focus there, but also work on the rest of your body as well.

How to Get Ripped Biceps Fast

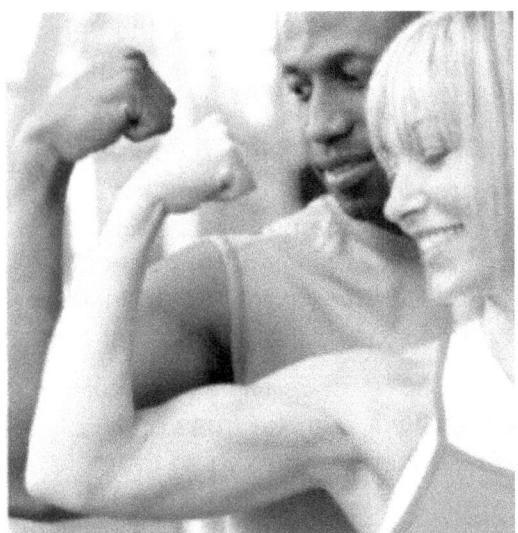

Increase arm strength with proper exercises.

When you talk to others about muscle building or strength
training, the first question is usually about how much he or she
can bring up.

While everyone wants strong abs, legs, and back muscles,
what you can "bring up" has a lot to do with your arm strength.
By doing the right kinds of arm workouts — along with
advantageous breaks from them — you can increase your
bicep muscle mass and strength. This way you can get ripped
biceps fast and begin asking everyone to the "gun show"!

Instructions: How to Get Ripped Biceps

Start by choosing a lighter weight than you would normally
want to use for lifting exercises. Try bumping 5 - 10 pounds

from the normal weights and note which muscles work harder as you do your lifts.

When using a heavier weight, other muscles such as the ambushes and deltoids catch the slack, meaning the biceps fon't have to work as hard. So use the lighter weights when trying to give your biceps a workout.

Break for 15 seconds between reps. This gives your biceps time to relax and replenish their oxygen stores which gives them the power to hold the pain associated with repetitions and gaining mass.

Also do some cardio every day. This is particularly good if you have body fat on your arms. Use a weighted jump rope which will give the biceps exercise while burning off that fat.

Compress every lift. When you're trying to get ripped biceps, you should compress the muscles tight at the top of every curl and keep it there for a few seconds.

Target the biceps only once per week. These muscles need to rest after a good workout and mend their tears. Allowing them time to heal is what helps them be able to build up mass.

Workout for How To Get Ripped Biceps

This is hard, but if you can deal with it you just might get whee you want to go.

BARBELL COILS -- Do 10 - 12 reps then super-set with ten dumbbell curls for another 10 - 12 reps. When you can't do any more reps on the tend curls do half reps, so only come up half the way.

By now your hands will barely be able to grasp but the longer you go the more benefit you'll get out of it.

The key here for getting ripped biceps is knowing how to get the most benefit from a single exercise. The longer the set endures, the more the body will break down -- meaning more fat burn.

So there you go. One of the best methods for burning fat and building up muscle at the same time!

However, to get the most benefit from your exercise program, you must also be eating properly.

Both. Diet and exercise. This is your answer for how to get ripped biceps.

What are the Best Chest Workout Exercises to Try?

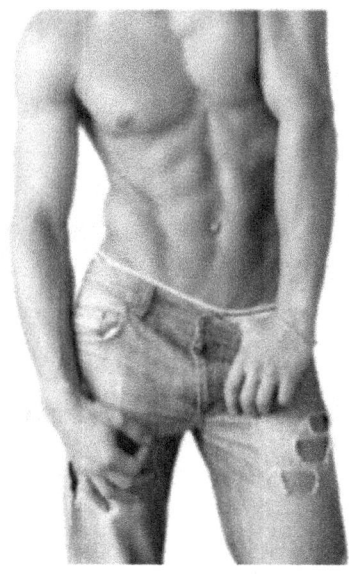

So you want to try some chest workout exercises but aren't sure about which would be right for you. Well, you should rest assured that there are a few in particular that will be really great for you. Some, even for females — but women don't tend to want their chest overly worked out.

Since men are more interested in increasing the definition of their pectoral muscles and learning about different chest workout exercises to try, the following ideas are for men.

Cable Crossovers Isolation Chest Exercise

A great chest workout exercise to start with is called cable crossover isolation chest exercise. This requires a special machine so it would probably be best to do this at your gym.

First, take hold of the handles that are attached to the overhead pulleys on your exercise machine. Make sure your arms are parallel to the floor. Now, with your palms down, bend slightly at the waist.

Next, bring your arms down in an arc movement until your hands meet. Then reverse the movement on your way back up to your original position.

Definitely, this is one of the best chest workout exercises you can try. After just a few reps of this exercise you **will** feel the burn. And when you get that feeling, you'll know you're that much closer to getting those really huge pecs that you want.

Dumbbell Pullover

You'll also want to try another great idea for a chest exercise: the dumbbell pullover.

This is a very easy exercise to do. Just remember to use a dumbbell instead of a barbell — which you would use if you were doing the bent arm barbell pullover.

To begin this exercise, lay face-up on a bench. Hold your dumbbell above your chest with your elbows slightly bent, then slowly lower the dumbbell so as to stretch you upper chest.

For the follow-through, you want to slowly lower the dumbbell back down over your head below the bench. This will give you a great stretch.

These are both great chest workout exercises to try but remember that these are only two of the many that are available to you.

Isn't it good to know there's such a variety of exercises for the chest that you can do?

Side Effects of Creatine — are they harmful?

Do you ever watch ULTIMATE FIGHTING CHAMPIONSHIP or any other type of serious fighting or athletic event? If so, then you've probably heard of Creatine before. This is a chemical produced by your body's muscles when they are used and stretched and exercised. This is a body chemical that serious athletes are interested in – and you should definitely be interested, too.

Creatine is also a supplement, but it's nothing like steroids which are a type of drug. As a supplement, this white crystalline powder can be healthy for your body and will help you excel in your sport.

More than anything you're probably wondering if there are any harmful side effects of Creatine for someone who wants to take it as a supplement. So, if you *are* interested in learning about possible harmful side effects of Creatine, then you are definitely going to want to continue reading the following information.

About the Product

Creatine is a compound that is involved in the production of energy in your body and is also present in small amounts in the red meat and fish that you eat. There are a number of reasons that people will take extra Creatine in the form of a supplement. For people performing sports activities, research suggests that Creatine supplementation may help improve performance in high density, short duration activities such as weight lifting and sprinting.

Harmful Long-term Side Effects of Creatine

When considering the possibility of taking a Creatine supplement, many people wonder if there are any harmful side effects that they should be concerned about. The answer is no — as long as there are no harmful additives in the formulation. No studies have reported long-term harmful side effects of Creatine that you should be concerned about.

Just be careful when buying Creatine as a supplement and read the ingredients on the label. Some companies add caffeine as an energy booster to their Creatine. This is something you don't want as it can be harmful if taken at a high dose for an extended period of time.

Although there has been some dispute in the past about whether or not Creatine is dangerous to take, research seems to have proven that there are no harmful side effects as long as you do not take more than the recommended dosage. There are other products similar to Creatine, but this seems to be the best choice for someone who has decided that supplementation is the way to go.

Short-term Side Effects of Creatine

While there are no reports of long-term serious side effects that you need to worry about, there are a few short-term side effects that you're going to want to watch out for. A few of the more common short-term side effects include:
– gas and bloating
– loose stools
– diarrhea
– muscle weakness
– cramping
– kidney stones

You'll have to decide if the possible benefits outweigh Creatine's possible discomforts.

#

EXCERPT FROM: *How to Eat Healthy – foods to eat . . . foods to avoid* by Joyce Zborower

When food is plentiful, what constitutes

CONTEMPORARY MALNUTRITION

When a layperson hears the term 'malnutrition', we generally see in our mind's eye the picture of a person, child or adult, with rail-thin limbs, a swollen abdomen, and flies crawling all over his/her face and into the eyeballs. The person has no energy with which to raise their arm to shoo them away. However, this is only one side of malnutrition. The other is obesity. Both are deleterious. Malnutrition, therefore, can be defined as any significant nutritional deviation from that which promotes healthy bodily functioning.

Malnutrition of the body, i.e. the whole organism, begins with malnutrition of the individual cells that make up that body.

The current, traditional model for identifying malnutrition is:

Maltutrition: an insufficiency of one or more nutritional
elements necessary for health and well being
-- Primary Malnutrition -- Caused by
-- (1) unavailable foodstuffs (as in poor economy, drought, or
over population)
-- (2) when food is plentiful, by poor eating habits

Secondary Malnutrition -- Caused by failure of absorption of
essential nutrients
i.e. – the body cannot _use_ the nutrients that are available in the
foods
-- (1) as in diseases of the gastrointestinal tract, thyroid,
kidney, liver, or pancreas
-- (2) by increased nutritional requirements (growth, injuries,
burns, surgical procedures, pregnancy, lactation, or fever); or
-- (3) by excessive excretion (diarrhea)

This model needs to be revised to include under 'Primary
Malnutrition':
-- (3) when food is plentiful **but essentially devoid of natural
micro-nutrients.**

Micro-nutrients are the vitamins, minerals, phyto-chemicals,
flavinoids, etc. that are present in fresh, natural, unprocessed
foods. They are very delicate and are easily destroyed by heat,
refining, and other processing procedures as well as by some
agricultural practices.

Macro-nutrients are the fats, carbohydrates and proteins that provide the calories your body either stores as fat or uses for energy. They are very stable and not easily destroyed or altered.

When nutrition gurus talk about "nutrients", they are usually referring to the **macro-** variety – and this is where the confusion arises. Since natural food consists of BOTH micro- and macro-nutrients, and their functions in the body are very different, and you CAN eat one without the other (as in highly refined products), I think it is vitally important that professionals be very specific about which type of nutrient they're talking about.

What is the reasoning behind this proposed change?

From the beginnings of food cultivation, around 10,000 B.C., until 1840 A.D. when Liebeg introduced his NPK (nitrogen, phosphorous, potassium) theory of plant growth, the only foods (from among the hundreds of ingredients available) that were routinely consumed in the refined state (natural nutrient content either severely reduced or eliminated) were: refined sugar (dating from prior to 510 B.C.), refined white wheat flour (dating from prior to 150 B.C.), and refined olive oils, another ancient practice. The production of olive oil began around 5,000 B.C., but I have not yet found a definitive date for when it began to be widely used as a refined product. These were, and are, staple foods.

When these were the primary natural micro-nutrient deficient foods consumed on a regular basis, the impact to the nutrition of the cells was low. (Food preservation, another ancient practice, also somewhat reduced natural micro-nutrient content but not nearly as severely as refining.) The ingestion of a greater majority of untreated, micro-nutrient-rich foods has the effect of "making up for" the nutrient deficiencies of the treated foods.

It is postulated that sugars entering the cells that do not contain sufficient natural micro-nutrients to adequately nourish the cells and provide energy for the work that the cells must do to sustain health and life causes the cells to suffer minute, discreet, cumulative damage that, over time, results in the overt symptoms of what we now call a food related disease.

Food related diseases are: cancer, hyper-tension (high blood pressure), kidney disease, heart disease, obesity (which is not really a disease), diabetes, stroke, and high cholesterol (which I also don't consider to be a disease).

Historically, only the most genetically susceptible individuals exhibited overt symptoms of food related disease, i.e. diabetes and kidney disease -- both ancient diseases.

With the advent of chemical agriculture, the micro-nutrient value of all foods produced by this method was slightly reduced. As these foods were fed to animals that were used as food, the micro-nutrient value of those foods for those of us higher on the food chain was also reduced slightly. (Do you see how this is becoming negatively cumulative?)

# # #

This is the end of this excerpt.

Check out: *How to Eat Healthy – foods to eat . . . foods to avoid* at Amazon.com

DISCLAIMER

This book is presented solely for informational and educational purposes so you can learn more about the subject.

The information provided in **Ab Workouts for Hardgainers** is NOT INTENDED TO PROVIDE MEDICAL ADVICE OR TREAT OR CURE ANY DISEASE OR HEALTH PROBLEM OR OFFER ANY SPECIFIC DIAGNOSIS TO ANY INDIVIDUAL. You should always consult your licensed healthcare professional before making significant changes to your diet or taking any form of medication.

I am NOT a licensed healthcare professional. My background and degrees are in Clinical Psychology and Certified Professional Coaching. However, I have had college level training in biology, human physiology and nutrition and have done extensive independent research in nutrition.

While I have made significant effort to provide accurate information, the information provided here should NOT be considered complete and exhaustive of the topic and I DISCLAIM ANY LIABILITY OR LOSS IN CONNECTION WITH YOUR USE OF THE INFORMATION CONTAINED HEREIN. YOUR USE OF ANY INFORMATION PROVIDED HERE IS TOTALLY YOUR RESPONSIBILITY.

You should never disregard medical advice or delay in seeking it because of something you have read here. This information is not intended as and should not be used in place of a visit to or consultation with or the advice of a physician or other qualified health care provider.

Questions and Comments?

We'd love to hear your thoughts.
Email us at admin@hunting4clients.com

One Last Thing Before You Go. . .

If you believe the book is worth sharing, would you take a few seconds and let your friends know about it on Facebook and Twitter? If it turns out to make a difference in their lives, they'll be forever grateful to you.

As will I.

All the best
Mike Weston/Joyce Zborower

or . . . If you enjoyed this book or found it useful, we would be grateful if you would post a short review on Amazon. Even just one or two sentences would be appreciated. They help other readers find our books.

Your support really does matter and we do read all of our reviews in order to make our books better. Just go to Joyce's Amazon page: http://amzn.to/MlKKpJ

Click the book cover to get to the 'Review This Book' button. Thank you for your support.

Amazon Top 3 Bestsellers in Ab Workouts

(3/31/2014)

1.

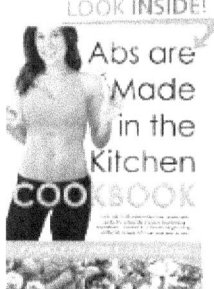

Abs are Made in the Kitchen Cookbook
By Christina Carlyle

2.

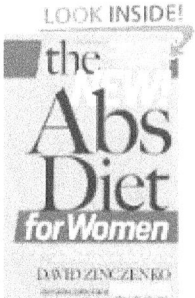

The New Abs Diet for Women
By David Zinczenko

3.

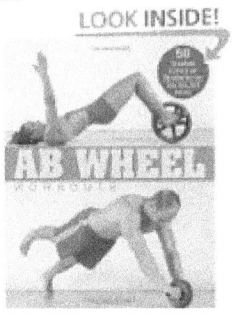

Ab Wheel Workouts
By Karl Knopf, M.D.

Recommended Books by K Pub Books

-- *YOUNG ADULT ROMANCE BOOKS* (no erotica) – by Sara Ann Nichols

Running Mates – a love story by Sara Ann Nichols

Destiny – a love story by Sara Ann Nichols -- Coming

-- *HEALTH & FITNESS/EXERCISE BOOKS* – by Michael Weston

Ab Workouts For Skinny Guys Who Want To Build Some Muscle and Turn Some Heads Even If You've Never Been Able To Do That With Other Workout Programs ---- by Michael Weston

Basic Ab Workouts Give You Sexy Flat Abs --- by Michael Weston

-- *MYSTERIES/SHORT STORIES* – by Joyce Zborower

The Trust – a cautionary tale

Little Mysteries – a short story

-- *CRAFTS BOOKS* – by Joyce Zborower

Handcrafted Jewelry Step by Step – 6 intermediate and advanced original designs

Handcrafted Jewelry Photo Gallery – cast jewelry -- fabricated jewelry

Wire Jewelry Photo Gallery – Original designs

Creations in Wood Photo Gallery – jewelry boxes, screens, storage ideas

Bargello Quilts Photo Gallery – quilt wall hangings

Bargello Train Quilt – cutting and sewing instructions

Sell Your Work – how to turn your craft into your business

-- FOOD/NUTRITION RELATED BOOKS – by Joyce Zborower

No Work Vegetable Gardening – for in-ground, raised, or container gardening

How to Eat Healthy – foods to eat . . . foods to avoid

The Truth About Olive Oil – benefits, curing methods, remedies

External Uses of Extra Virgin Olive Oil – Folk Remedies ... Body Lotions ... Pet Treatments

Signs of Vitamin B12 Deficiencies – Who's at Risk – Why – What Can Be Done

13 Easy Tomato Recipes – nature's lycopene rich superfood for heart health and cancer
protection

3 Fruit Pie Recipes – apple, cherry, crisp persimmon

BBQ Spare Ribs Recipe – with homemade honey BBQ sauce

Paleo Slow Cooker Recipes – by Julie Anderson

-- PSYCHOLOGY BOOKS – by Joyce Zborower and/or John F. Walsh

Psychology of Success – how to have success when trying to change how you look

Different Types of Depression – Characteristics and Treatments by Joyce Zborower and John F. Walsh

How to Fight Depression – 9 case studies ---- by John F. Walsh

Clinical Psychology – A Professional Perspective – memoirs and experiences – John F. Walsh

-- CHILDREN'S BOOKS – by Joyce Zborower

Baby Pics Counting and Number Book -- 1-13 The numbers are in numerals and words with lots of photos of babies.

Christmas ABCs – cute animal illustrations

Most of the above are also available as print-on-demand paperback editions. Also:

Grandma's No Work Vegetable Gardening – (paperback edition) same as *No Work Vegetable Gardening* except the photos are B&W and the price is lower.

-- Español Libros (Spanish language Books)

-- by Joyce Zborower and M. Angelica Brunell S.
Haga click aquí para ir a mi página de Amazon --
http://amzn.to/MlKKpJ
Pequeños Misterios – cuento
Joyas Artesanales Galeria de fotos – Joyas fundidas – joyas forjadas
Joyas de Alambre - Galería de fotos – Diseños originales
Creaciones en Madera- Galería de fotos – joyeros, biombos, ideas de almacenaje
Quilts Estilo Bargello - Galería de fotos – tapices de quilt
Bargello Quilt de Tren – instrucciones para cortar y coser
Vende tu Trabajo – como transformar tu arte en negocio
Signos de deficiencia de vitamina B12 -- Quén esta en riesgo – Por qué – Qué puede hacerse
Huerto sin Esfuerzo – para jardinería en el suelo, elevada o en contenedor
La Verdad Acerca del Aceite de Oliva – beneficios, métodos de curación, remedios
3 Recetas de Pie de Fruta -- Manzana, Cereza, Caqui fresco
13 Recetas de Tomate Fáciles -- Superalimentos de la naturaleza ricos en licopeno para la salud del corazón y protección contra el cáncer
Receta de Chuletas de Cerdo en Barbacoa -- con salsa casera de barbacoa con miel
Fotos de Bebés Libro de Números y de Contar De 2 a 5 años – 1 – 13
ABCs de Navidad – Para niños de 2 a 5 años

-- Italian Language Books

La verita su olio de oliva ... Prestazoini – Metodi di polimerizzazione -- Rimidi

-- Other Recommended Books

The Confession of a Trust Magnate ----- by George Allen Yuille

*Picture the combined navies of the world
anchored off our seaboard cities, the
combined armies of the world in possession
of our inland cities, envoys from each
nation congregated at Washington
partitioning our country, the entire population
being apportioned as slaves to do the bidding
of the conquerors.*

Would you be interested?

*An equally appalling situation confronts
the people of this country to-day.*

Read of it in the pages of this book.

This book was written in 1911. Its message is critical for today – 2014.

Ab Workouts for Skinny Guys Who Want to Build Some Muscle and Turn Some
Heads Even If You've Never Been Able to do That With Other Workout Programs